DO YOU WANT TO BE A

VETERINARIAN?

Coloring & Activity

Book

By Laura Halsey
DVM, cVMA

To the compassionate hearts and caring souls who make the world a better place for our furry friends,
This book is dedicated with immense gratitude to the animal lovers, whose unwavering love and kindness create a haven for creatures big and small. Your devotion to our four-legged companions is a beacon of light, bringing joy and comfort to their lives.

To the dedicated veterinarians, the unsung heroes of the animal kingdom, this dedication is a tribute to your tireless efforts, boundless compassion, and the countless lives you touch. Your commitment to the well-being of animals is a source of inspiration, and we honor the invaluable contributions you make to their health and happiness.

To the supportive community surrounding our veterinary practices, thank you for embracing our mission and fostering a bond that goes beyond the clinic walls. Your trust, cooperation, and shared love for animals create a community that nurtures and uplifts.

May this book serve as a token of appreciation to all those who dedicate their lives to the well-being of animals, reminding us that together, we can create a world where love and care know no bounds and inspire the next generation.

With heartfelt gratitude,
Laura Halsey,
Veterinarian & Author

Embark on a Journey of Caring

Becoming a veterinarian is like going on an exciting
adventure filled with love and care for animals.

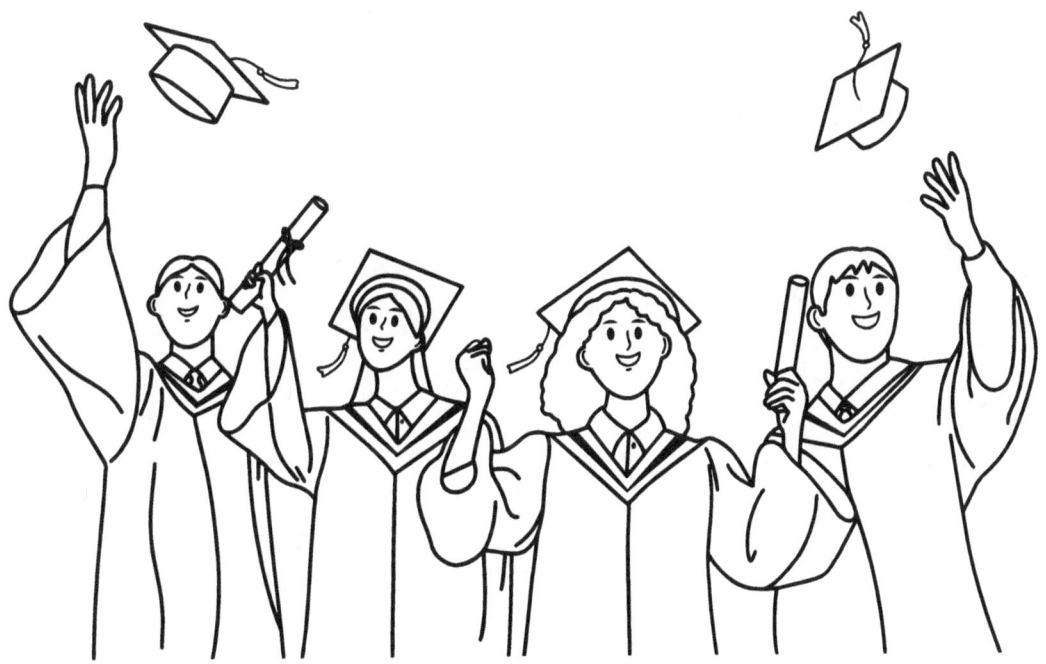

Veterinarians study chemistry, biology, and medicine.

Start

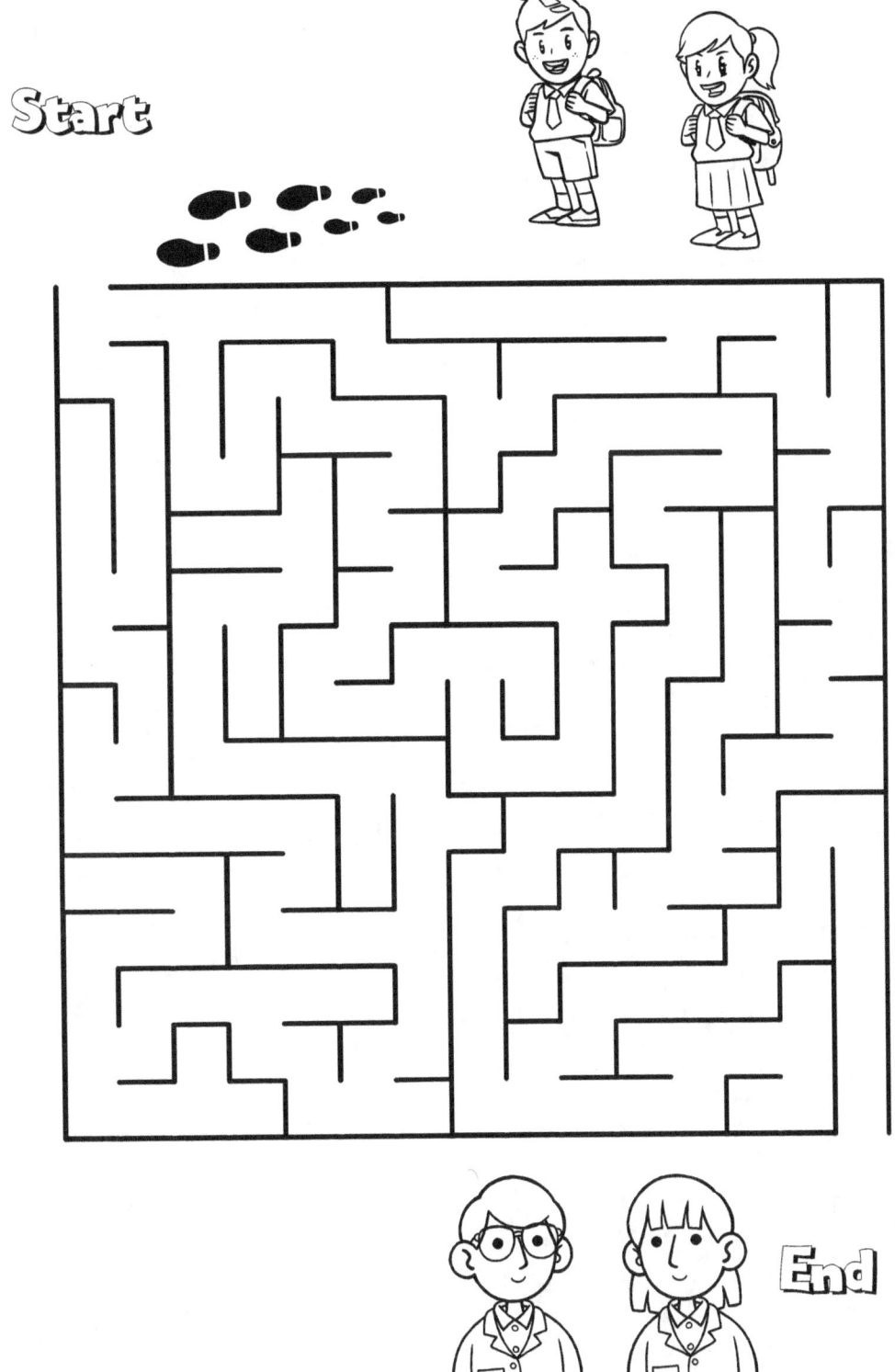

End

Helping Furry Friends

Veterinarians are like superheroes for animals, making
sure they stay happy and healthy.

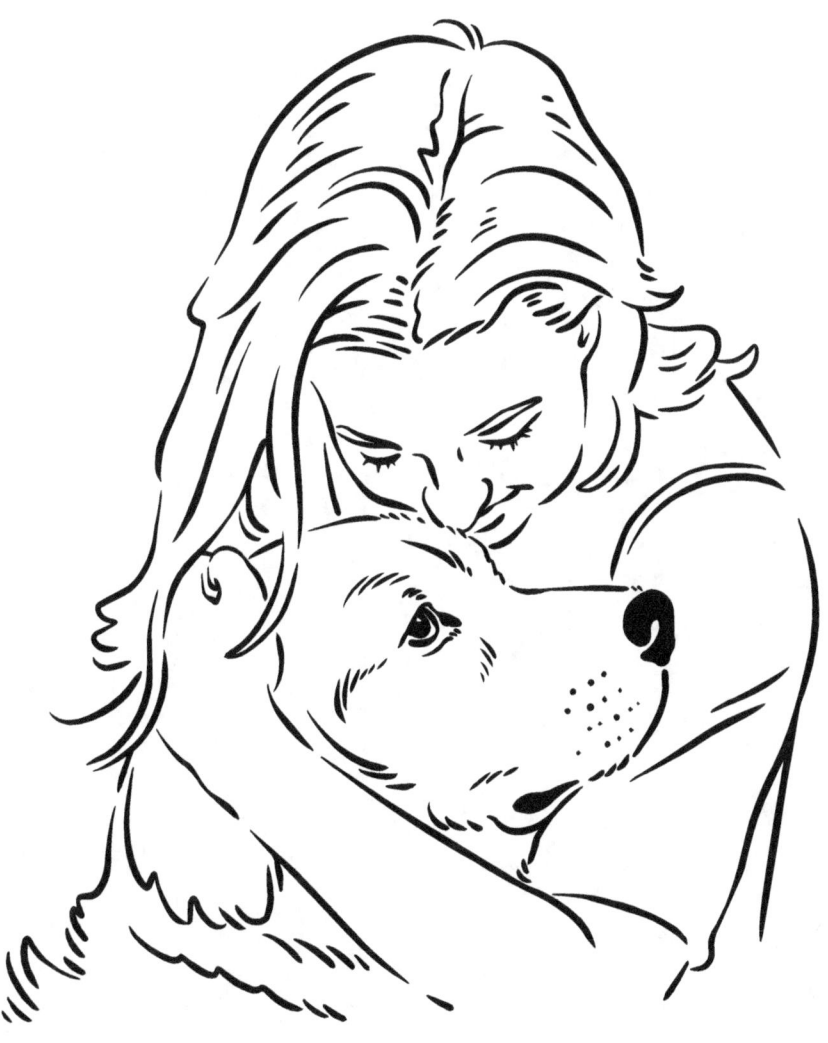

Find the

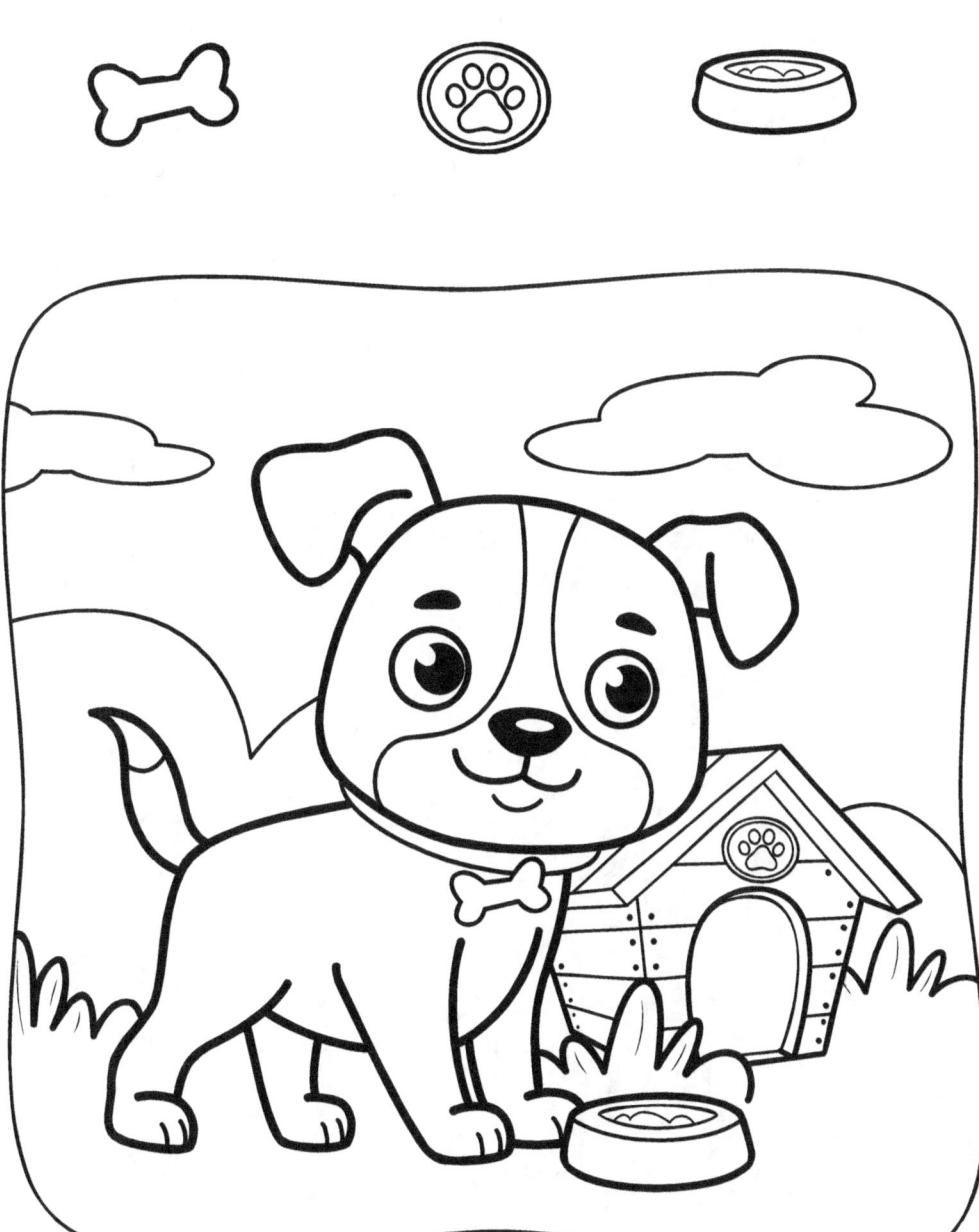

Animal Doctors

Just like doctors for people, veterinarians are doctors for animals, making sure they feel better when they're sick.

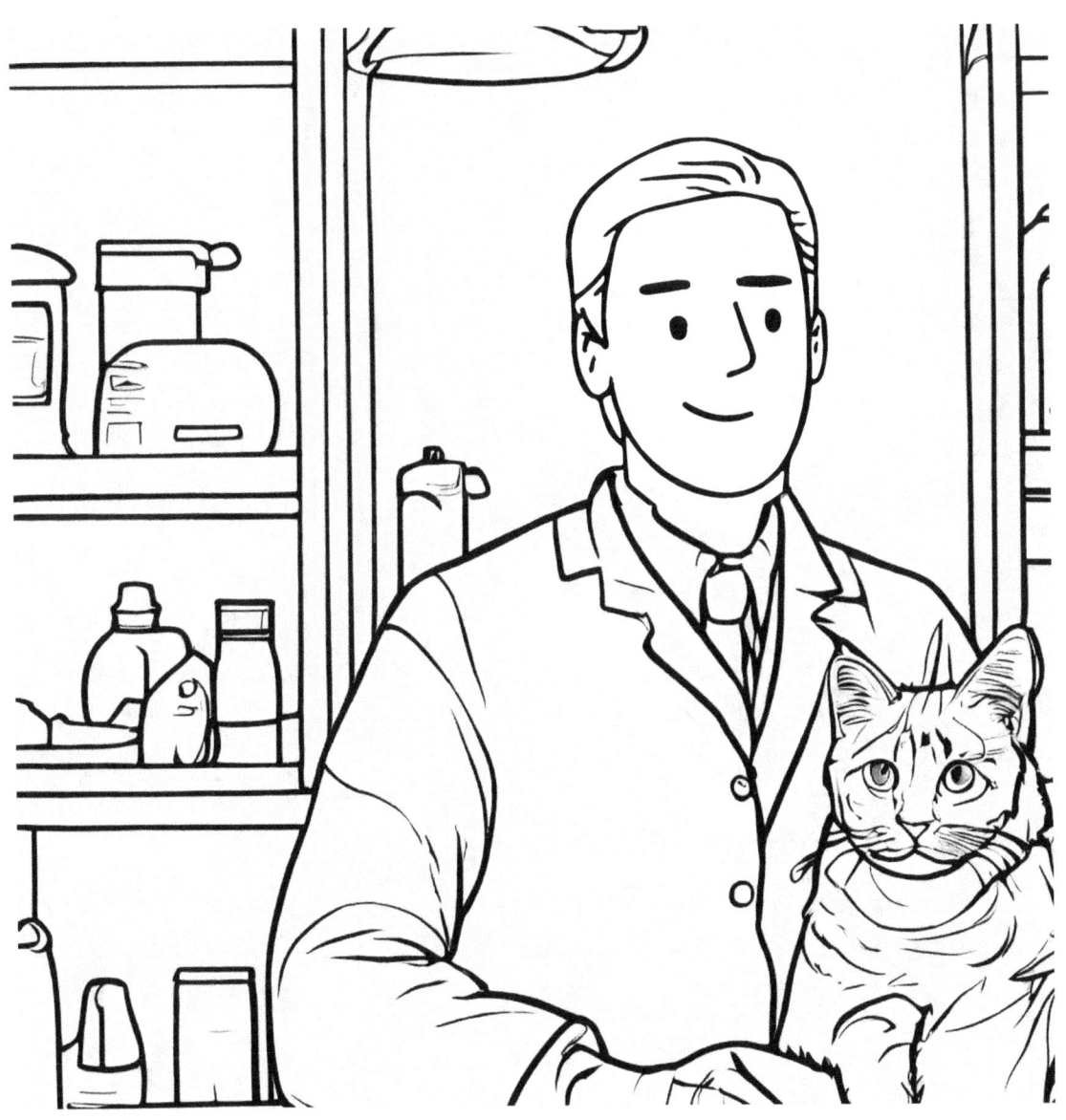

How Many Spots?

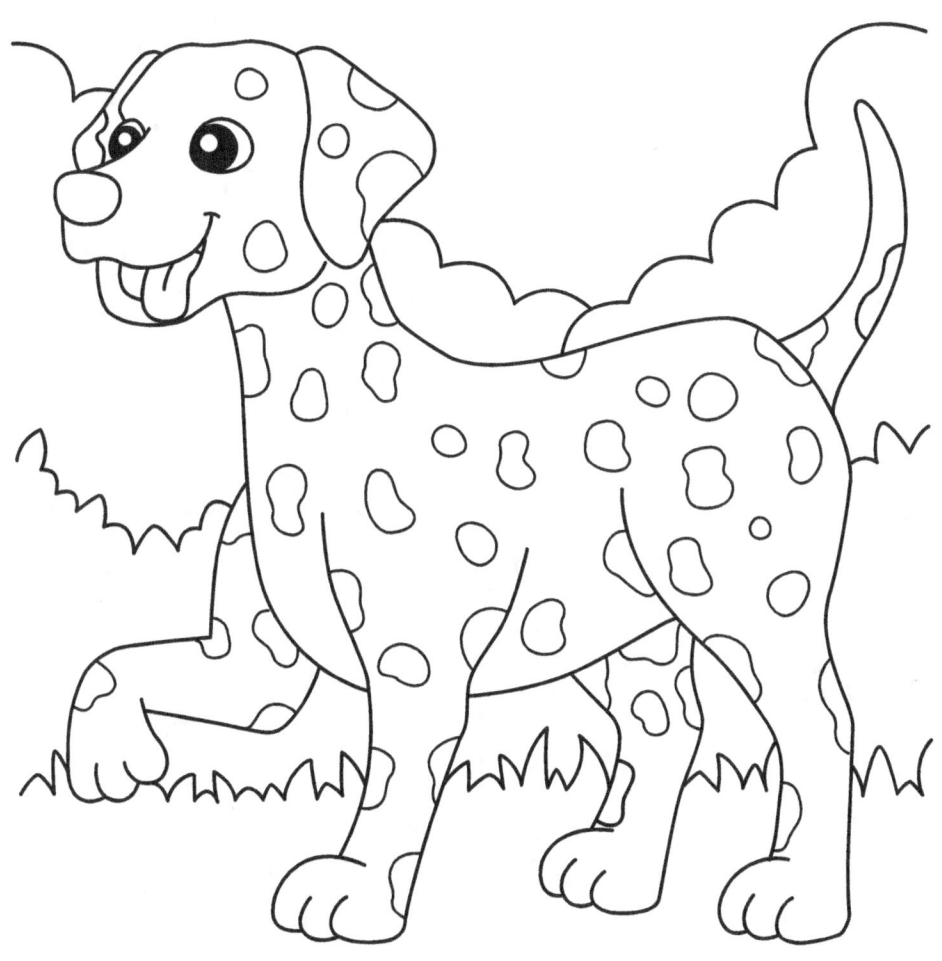

Watch and Learn

Veterinarians use all their senses. They must rely on their observations to learn what might be bothering animals.

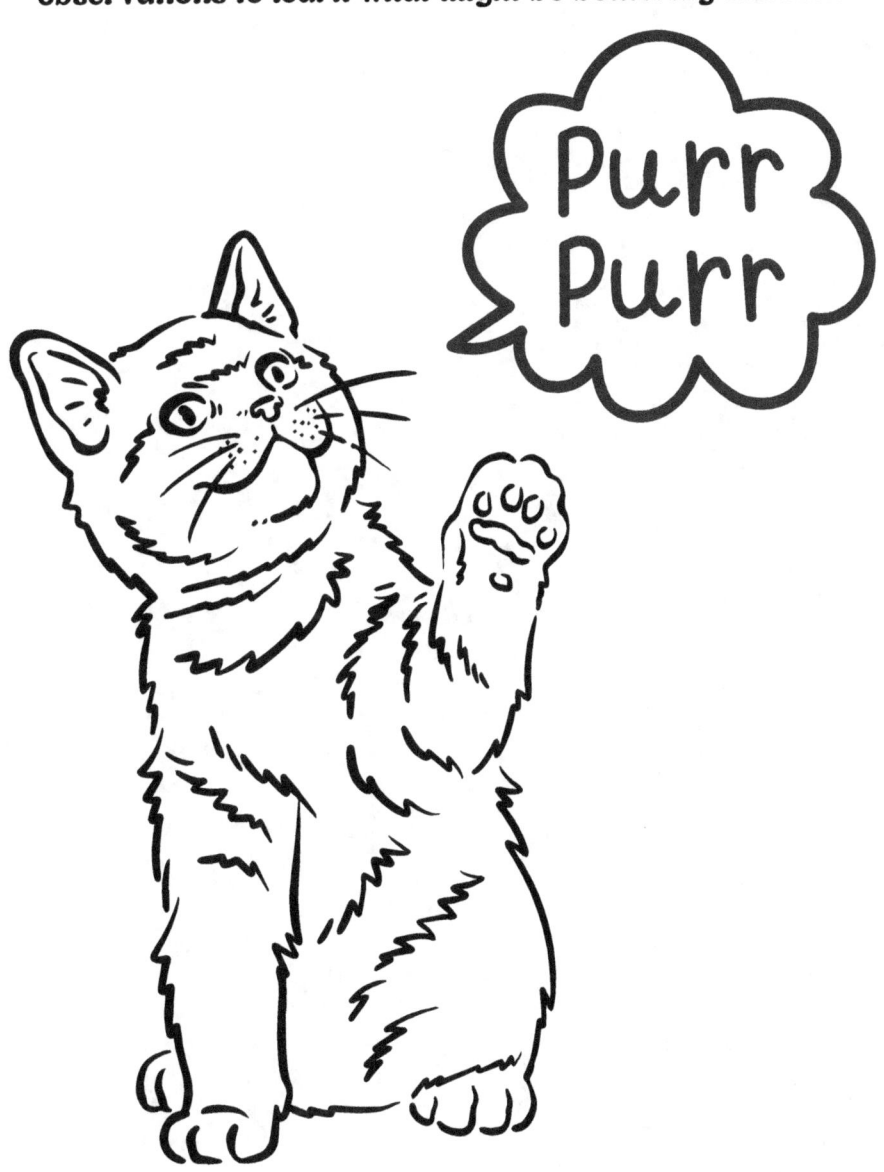

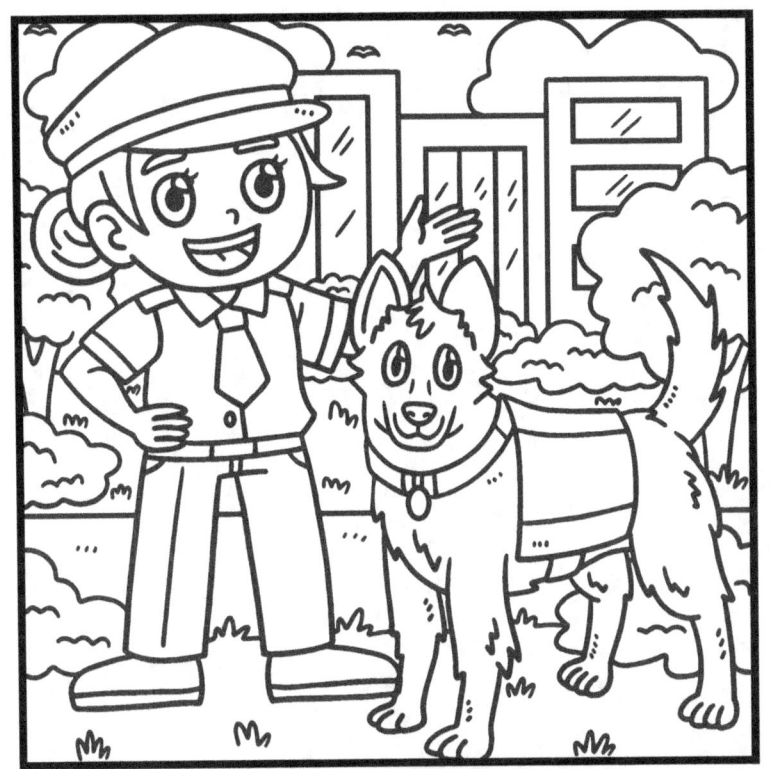

Find the 5 missing details

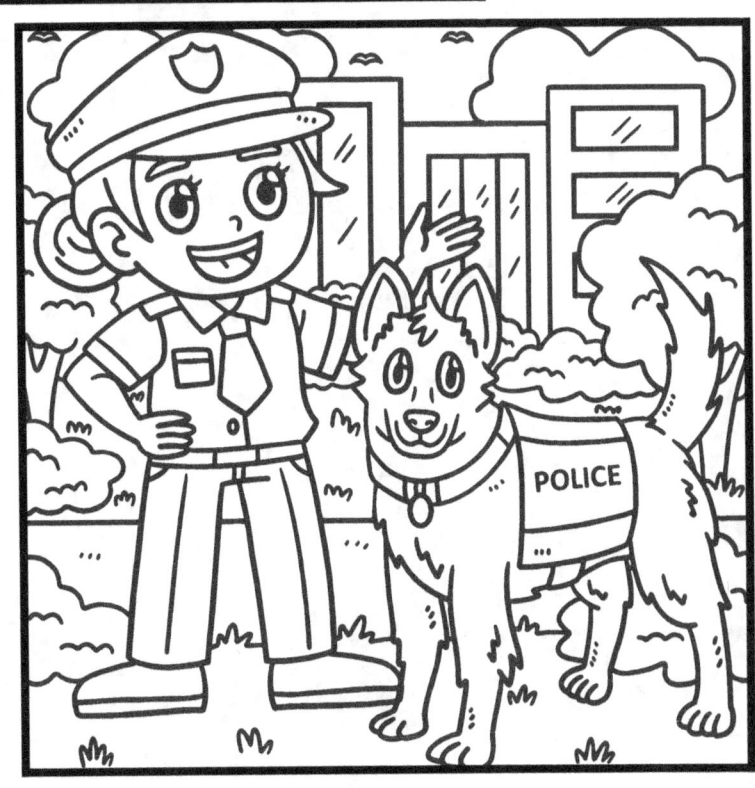

Furry Check-ups

Veterinarians perform exams on healthy animals to
screen for problems, including cute puppies and kittens, to
make sure they are growing up strong and playful.

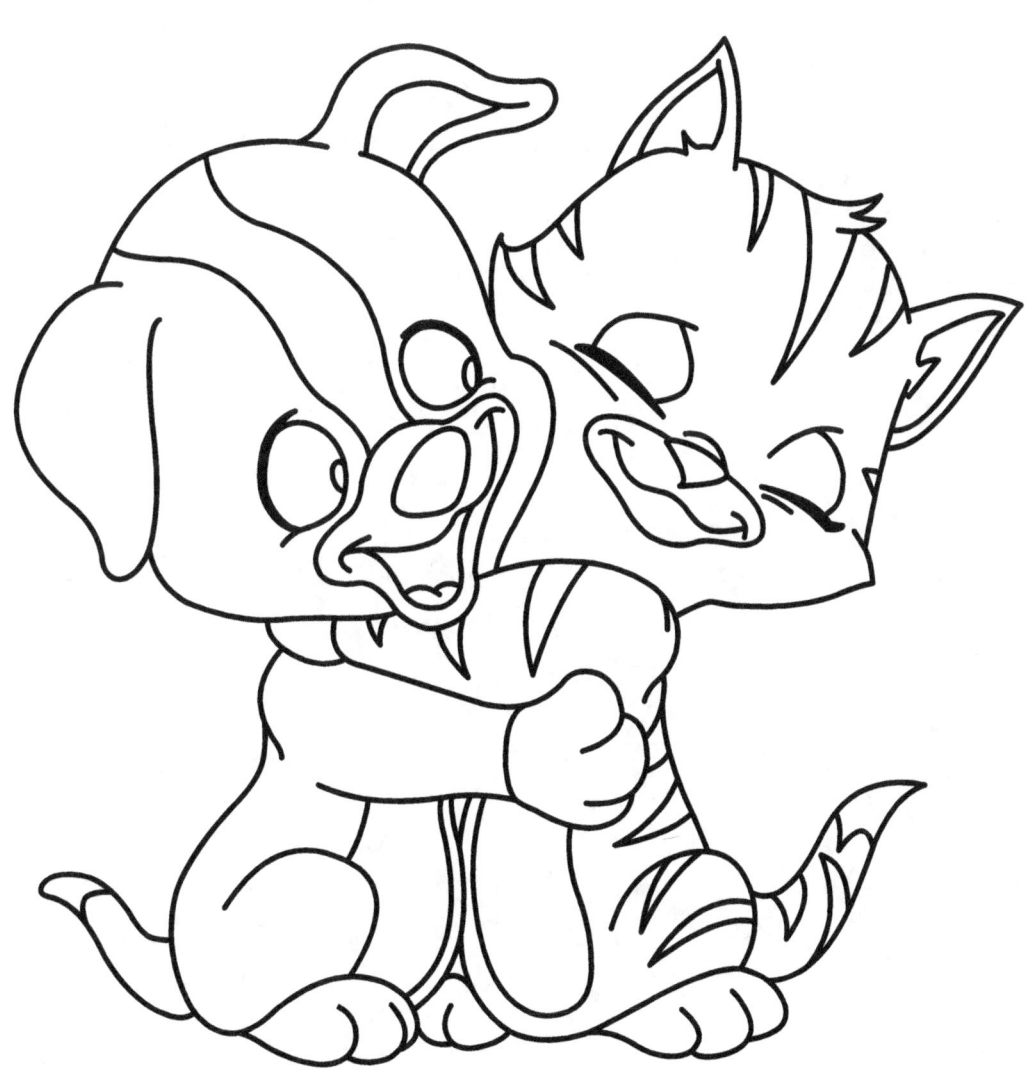

WORD SEARCH

DOG   CAT   RABBIT
HORSE   PIG   BIRD
VETERINARIAN   DOCTOR   SURGERY
FARM   GOAT   VACCINE

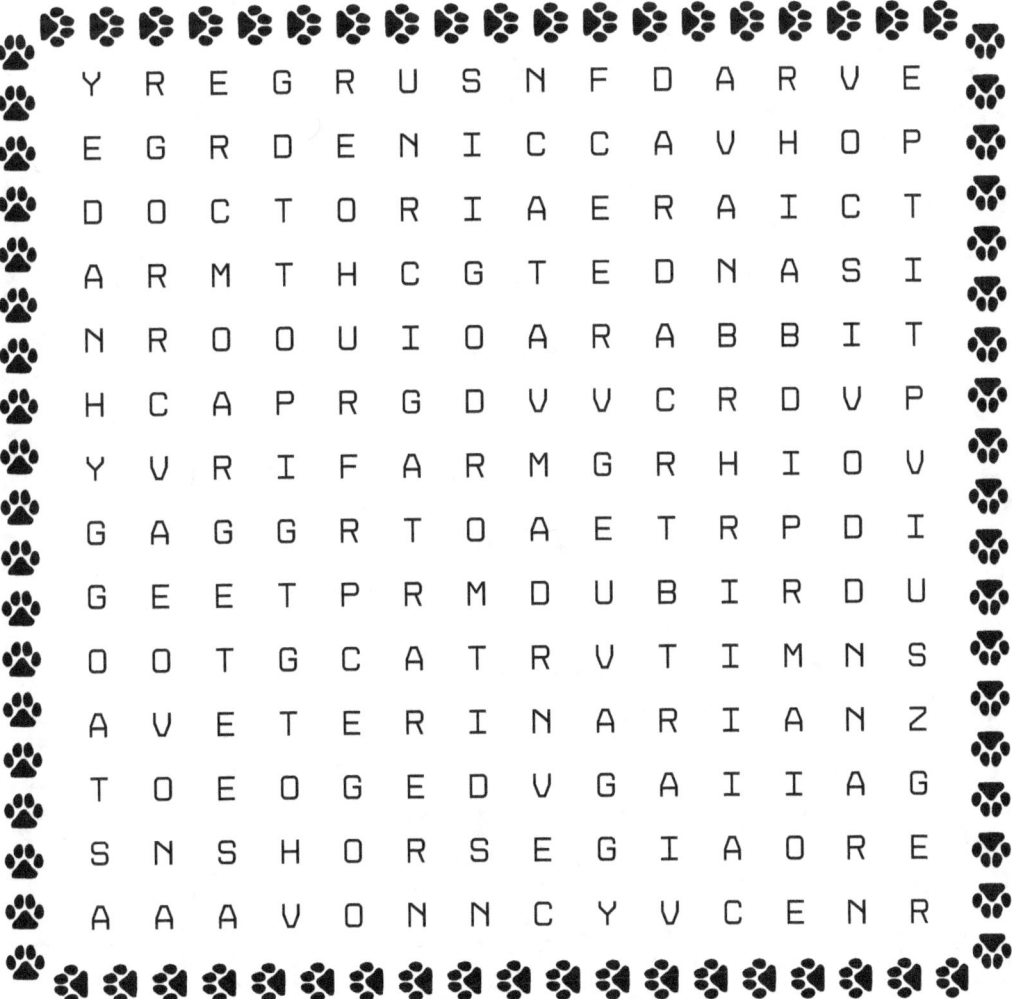

```
Y R E G R U S N F D A R V E
E G R D E N I C C A V H O P
D O C T O R I A E R A I C T
A R M T H C G T E D N A S I
N R O O U I O A R A B B I T
H C A P R G D V V C R D V P
Y V R I F A R M G R H I O V
G A G G R T O A E T R P D I
G E E T P R M D U B I R D U
O O T G C A T R V T I M N S
A V E T E R I N A R I A N Z
T O E O G E D V G A I I A G
S N S H O R S E G I A O R E
A A A V O N N C Y V C E N R
```

Animal Friends Everywhere

As a veterinarian, you get to meet all kinds of animals -
from fluffy pets to scaley reptiles!

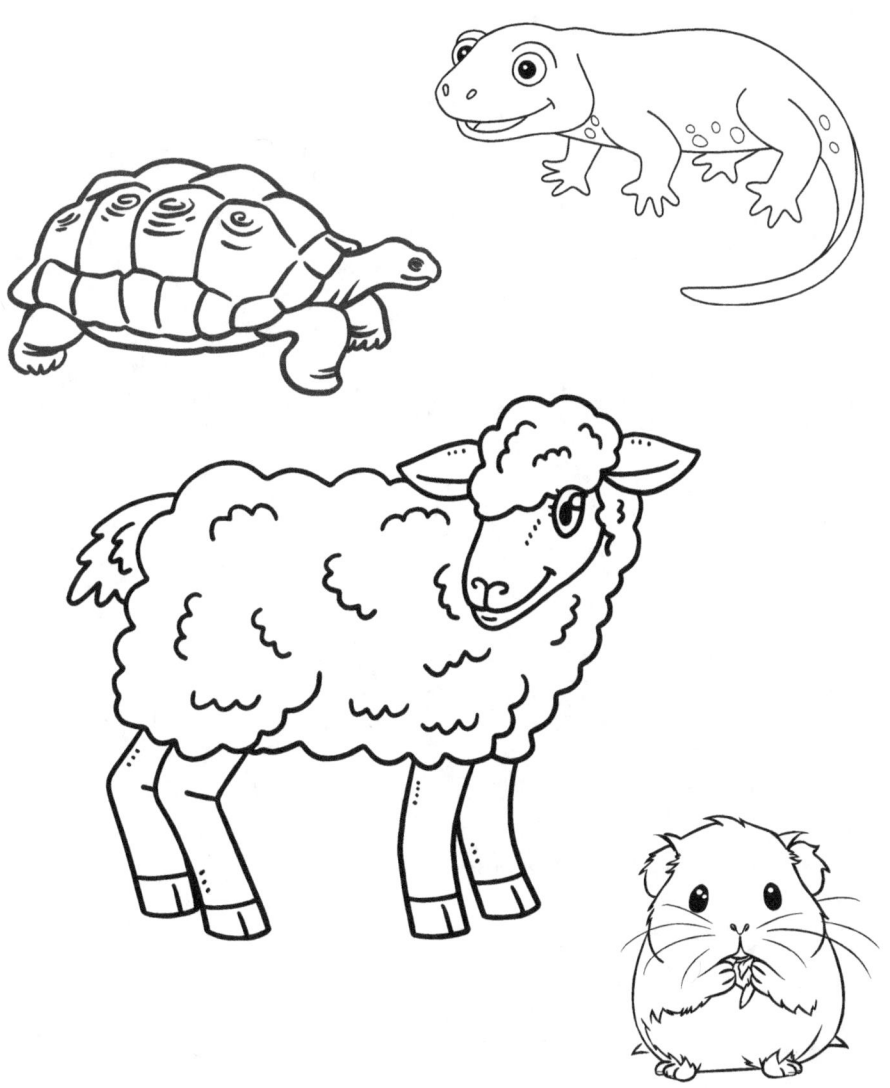

Match the Home

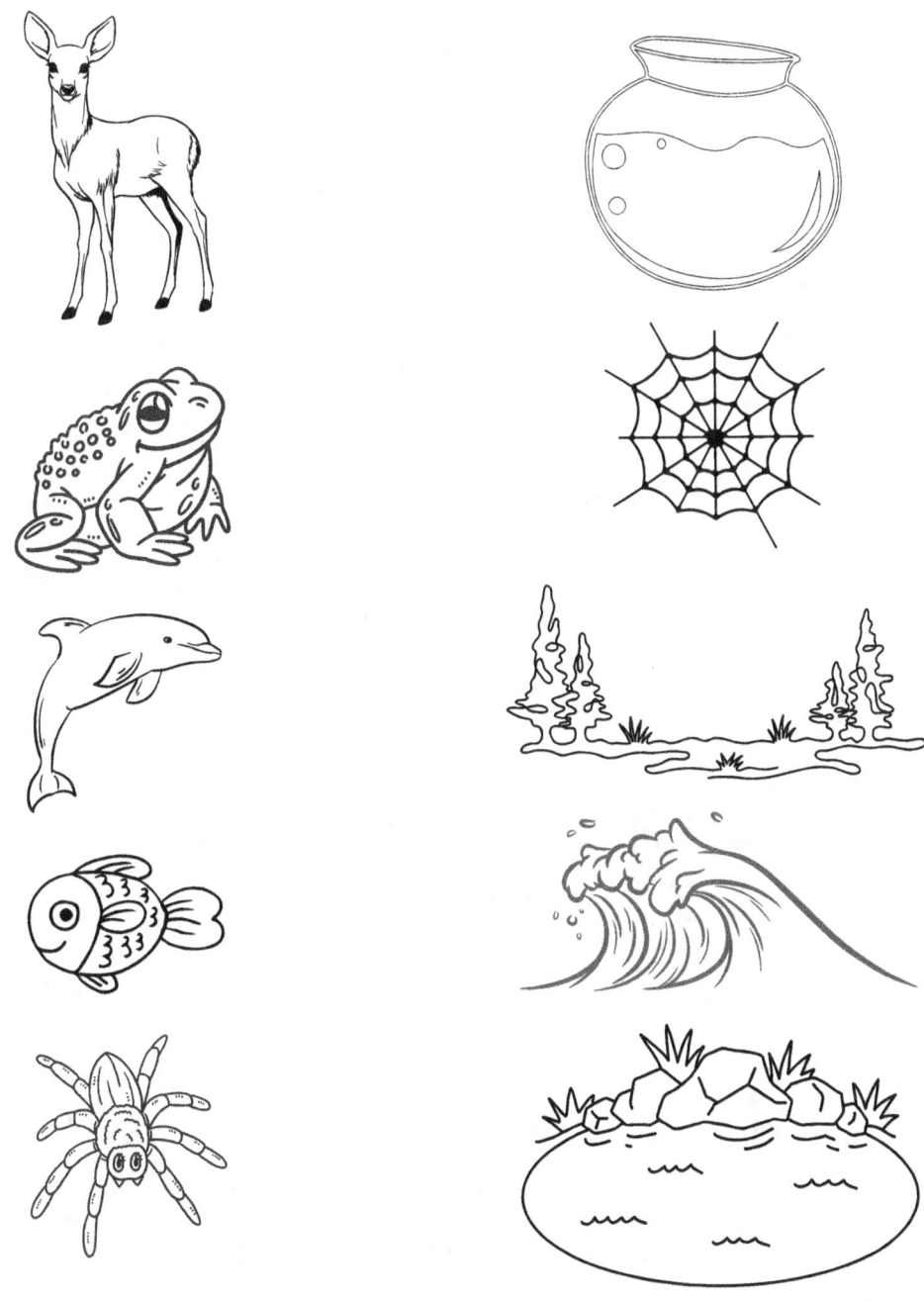

Solving Animal Puzzles

Vets are like detectives, figuring out what's wrong with an animal and finding the best way to help them.

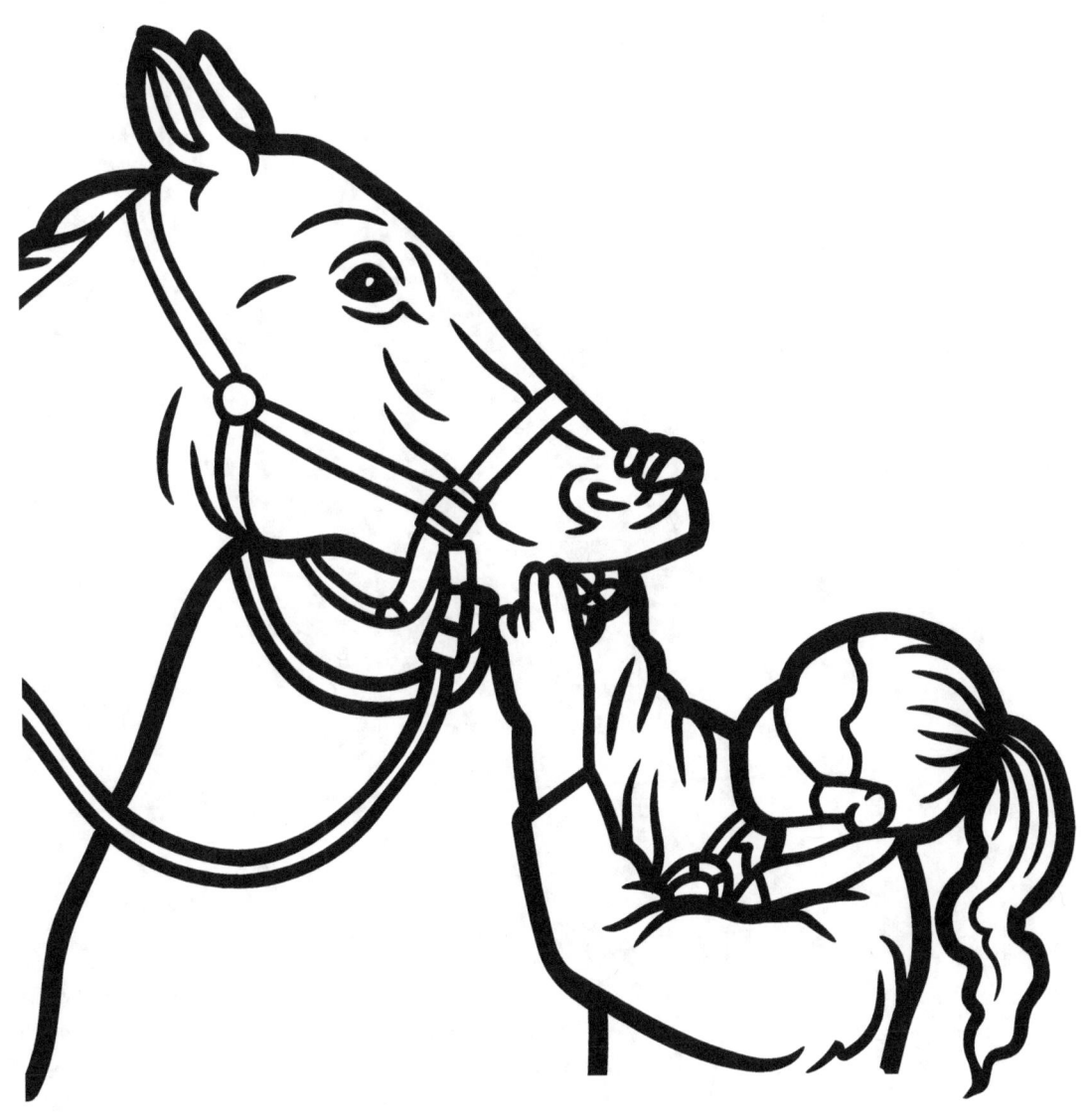

Help the puppy get the food bowl

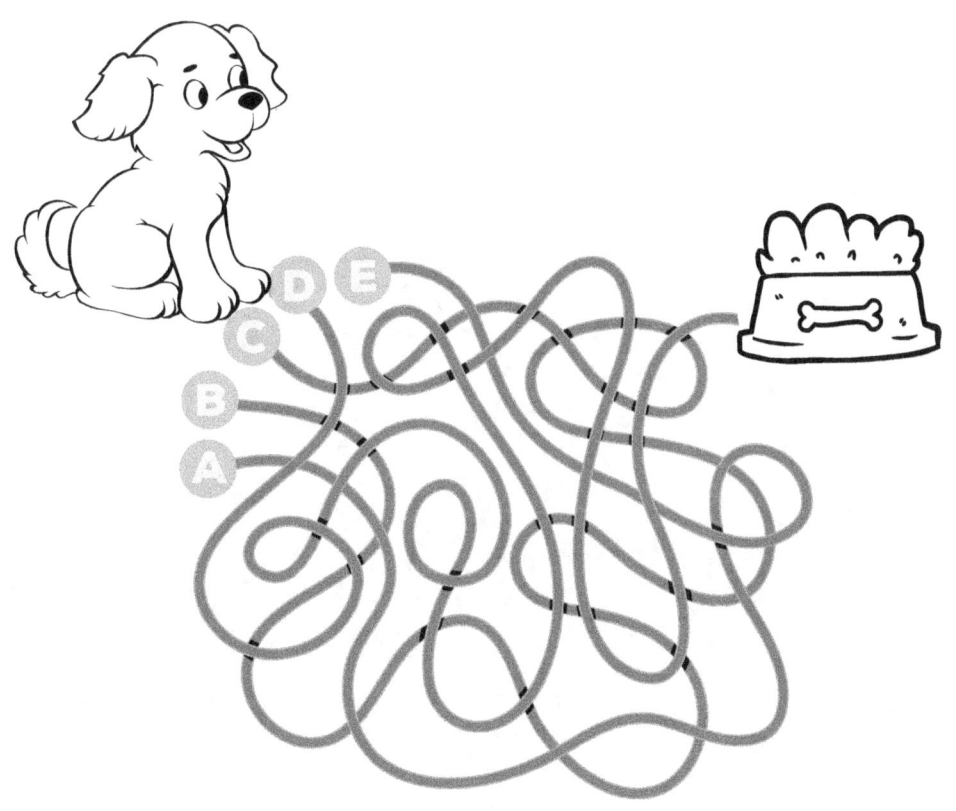

Kindness is Key

Veterinarians are super kind and caring; they treat every
animal with love, just like a best friend.

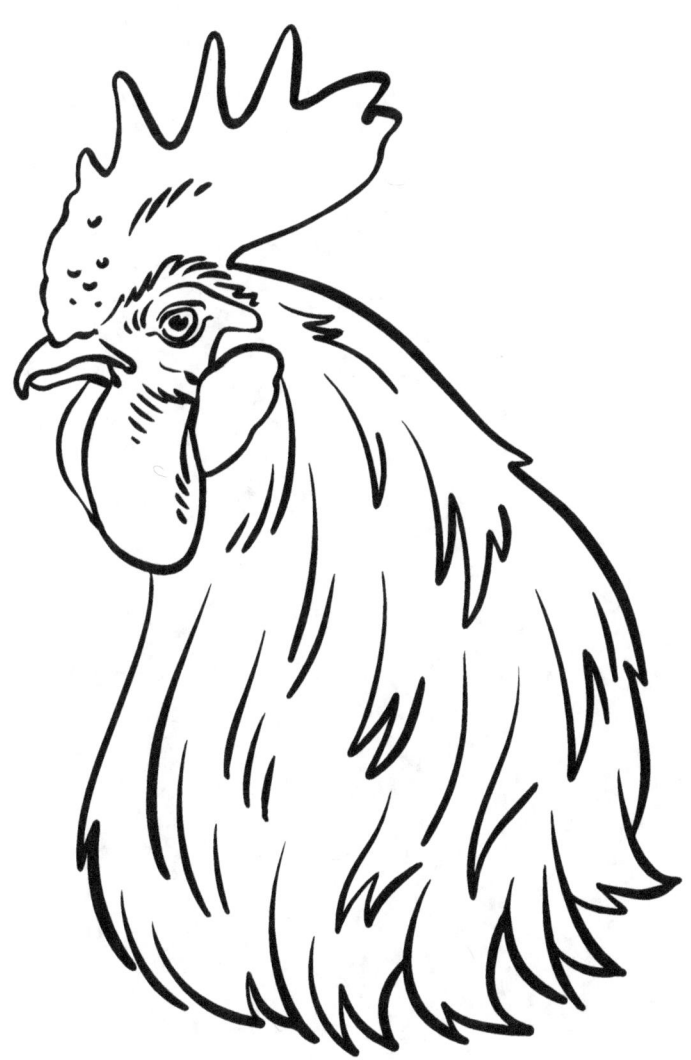

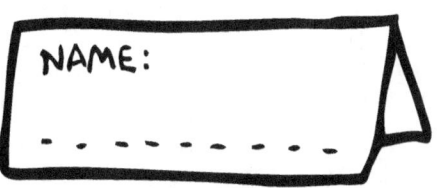

NAME:

- - - - - - - - -

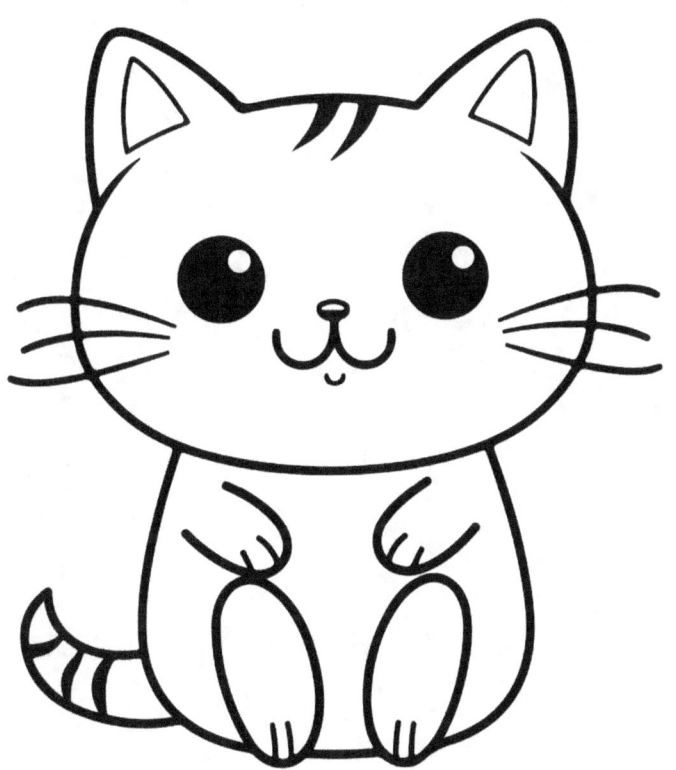

Name the kitten

Learning about Animals

To be a great vet, you'll get to learn fascinating things about different animals and how to keep them happy.

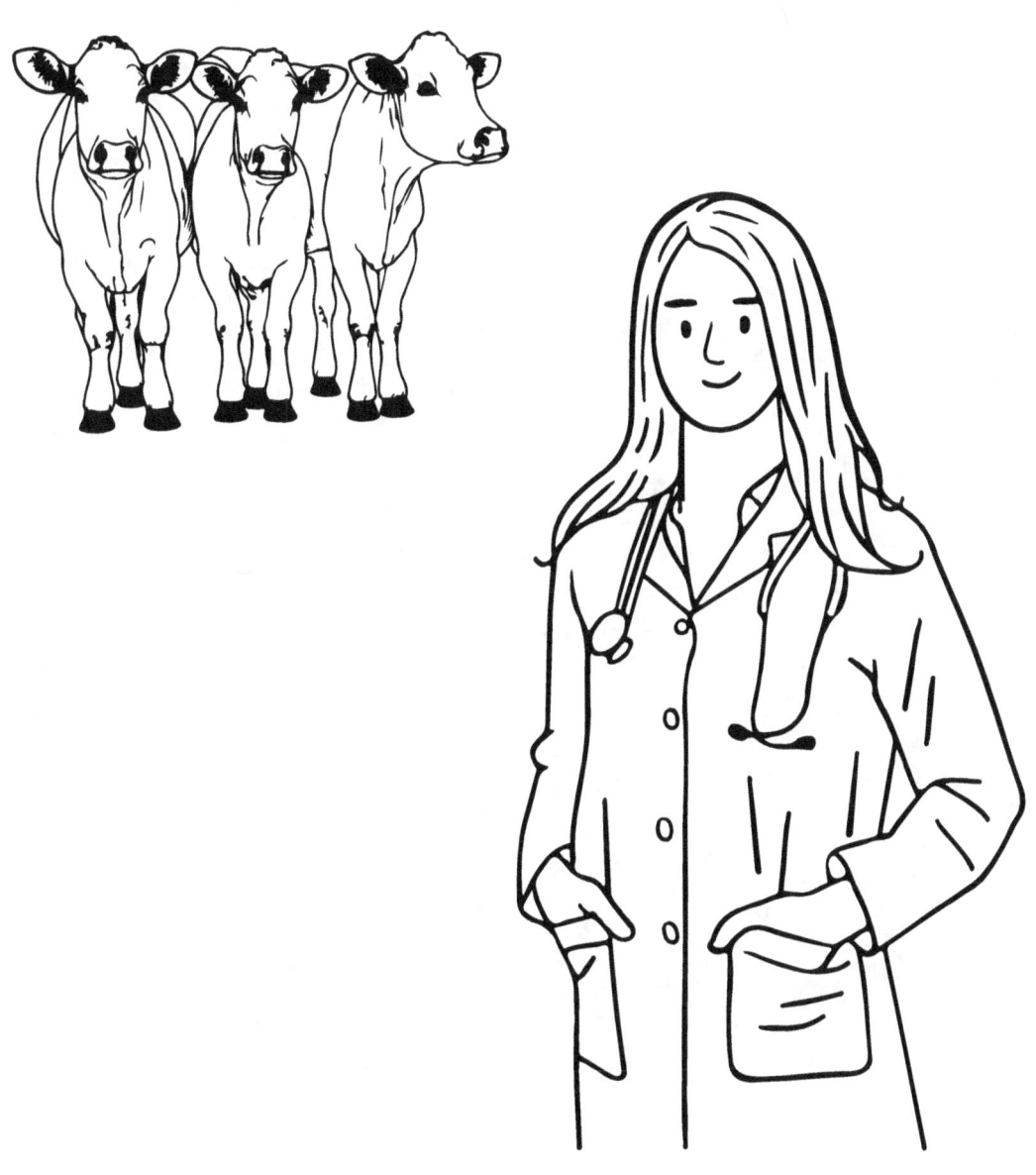

Word Scramble

WOBL   _ _ _ _

DOFO   _ _ _ _

MILANA   _ _ _ _ _ _

SAWP   _ _ _ _

OFOH   _ _ _ _

RABN   _ _ _ _

Saving the Day

Vets save the day by making sure animals stay safe,
strong, and ready for lots of fun

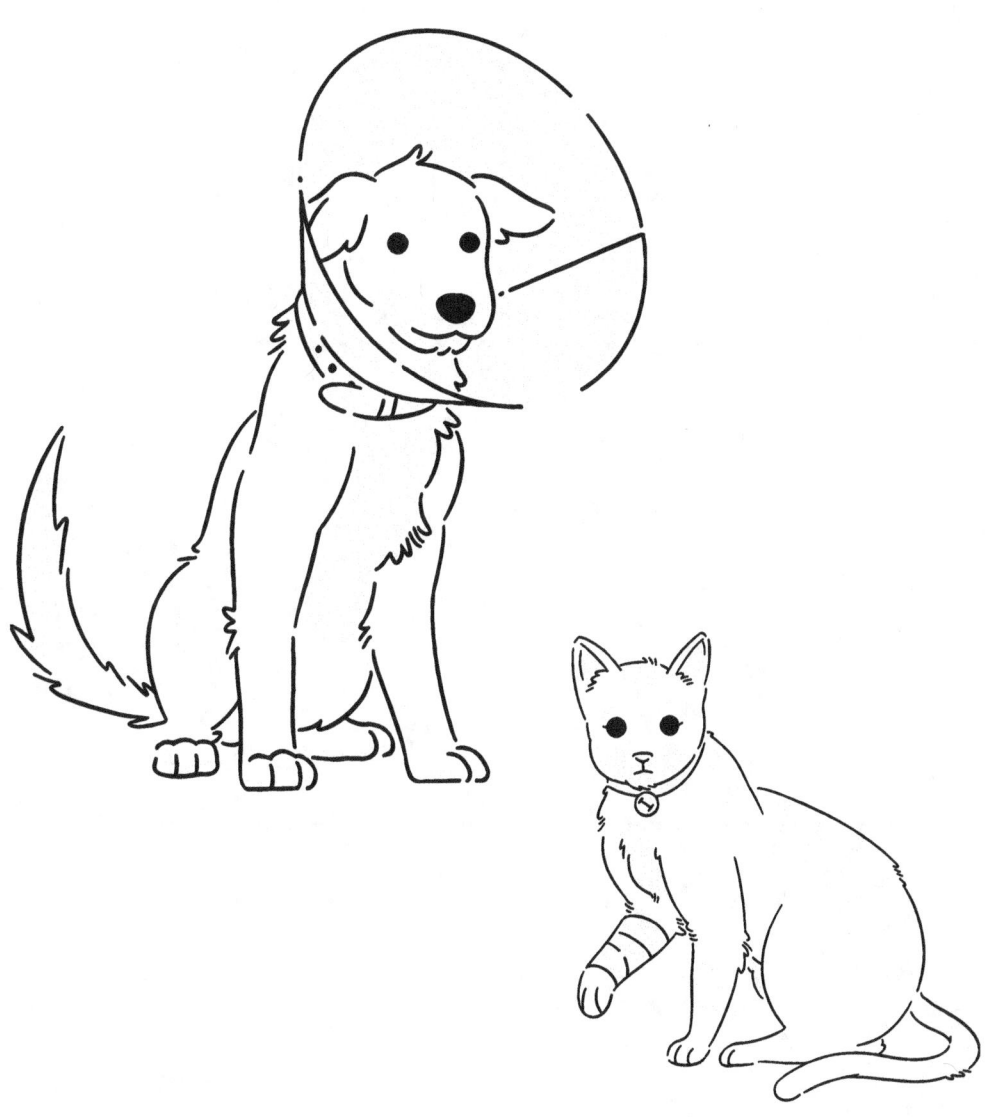

Find the 5 Items that Don't Belong

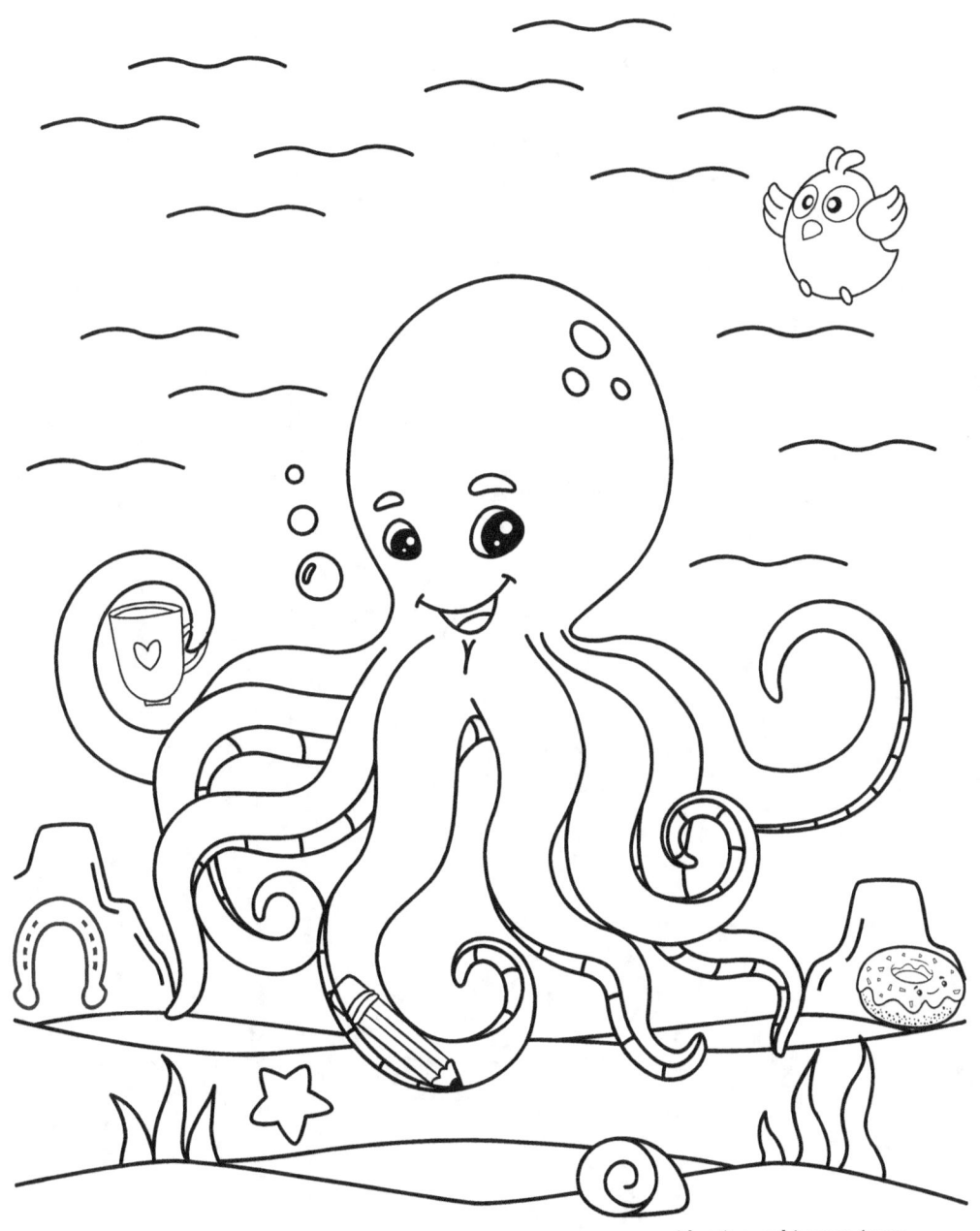

bird, donut, pencil, cup, horseshoe

Busy Vet Hospitals

Many veterinarians work in animal hospitals, making sure every patient gets the special care they need.

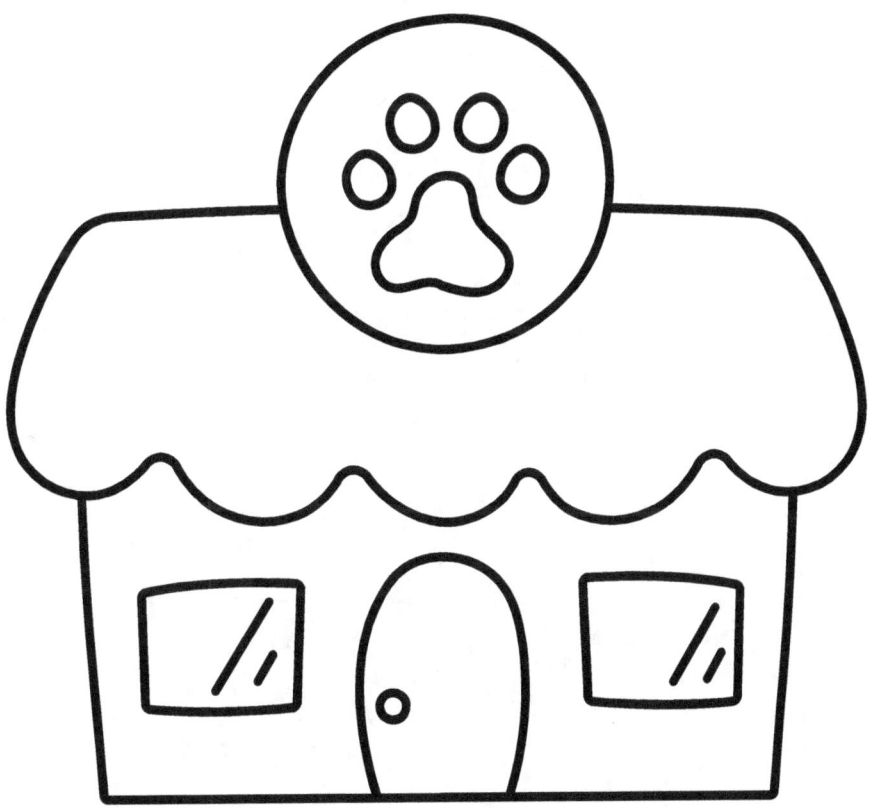

What would you name your vet hospital?

5. 6.
4.
7.
3.
8.
2.
18. 12. 11.
19. 10.
1. 20. 9.

.16 13.
15. .17
14.

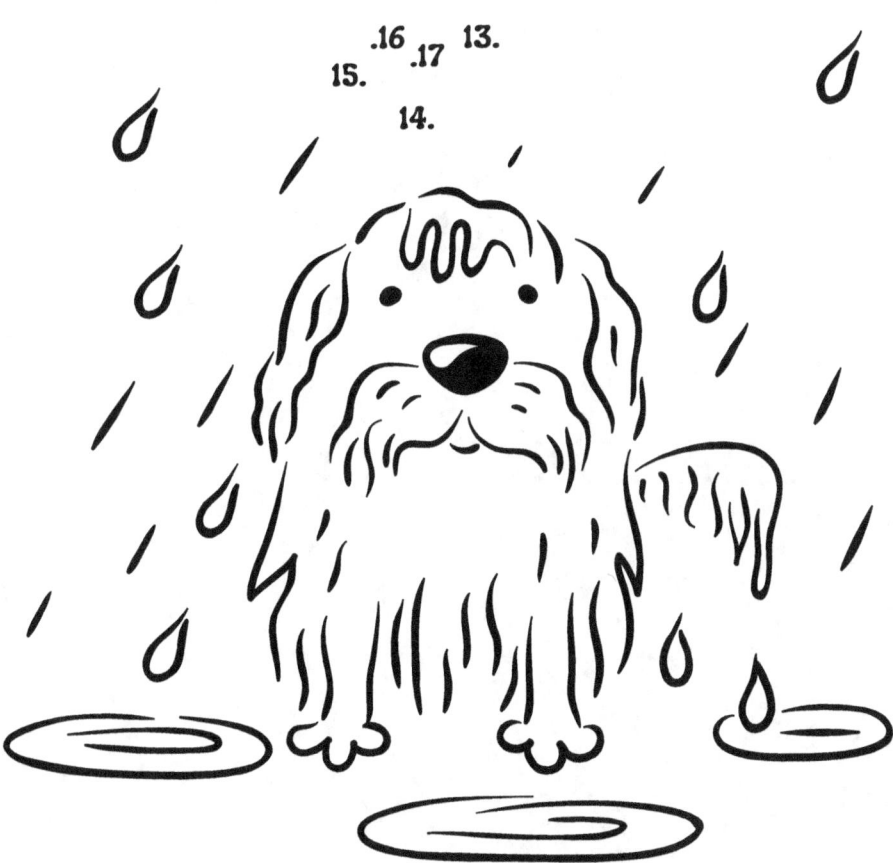

Connect the dots to stop the rain.

Many Ways to be a Vet

Veterinarians may work out of barns, on the road, in zoos, animal shelters, and more. Vets are also researchers, teachers, food safety inspectors, wildlife rehabilitators, and more.

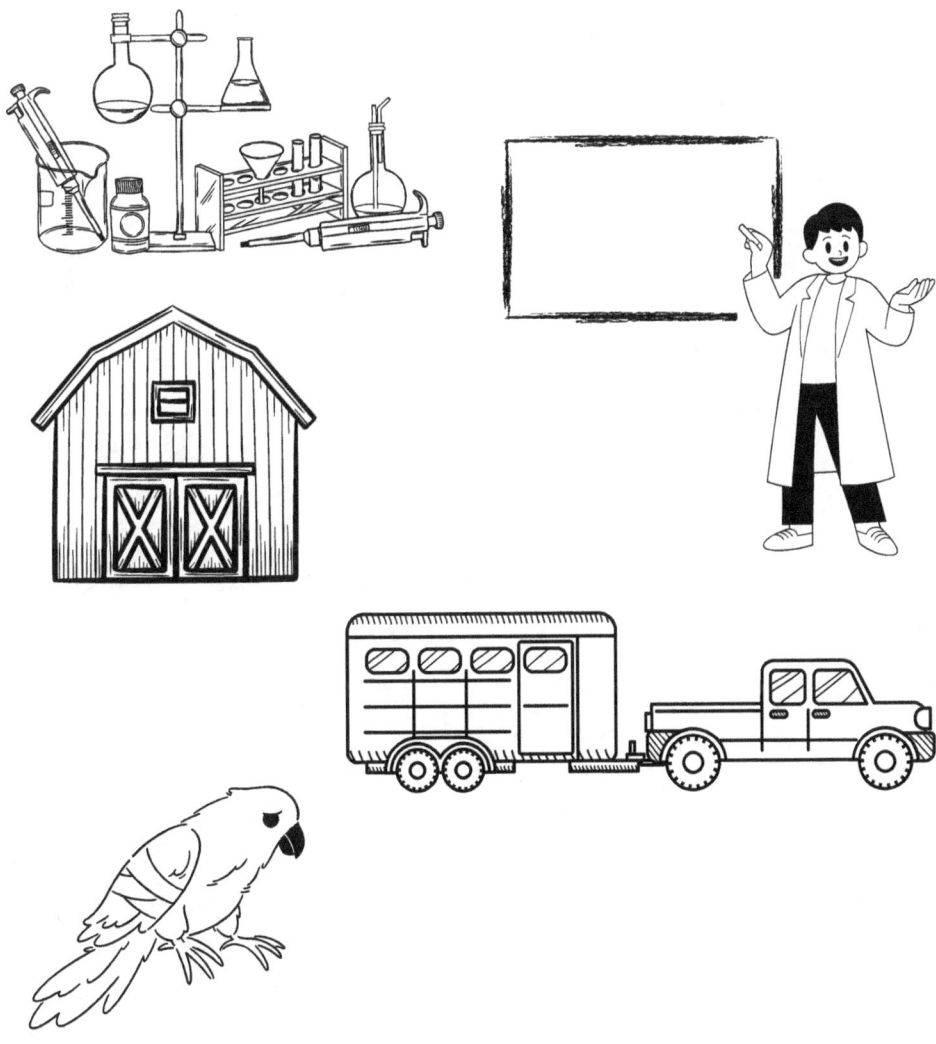

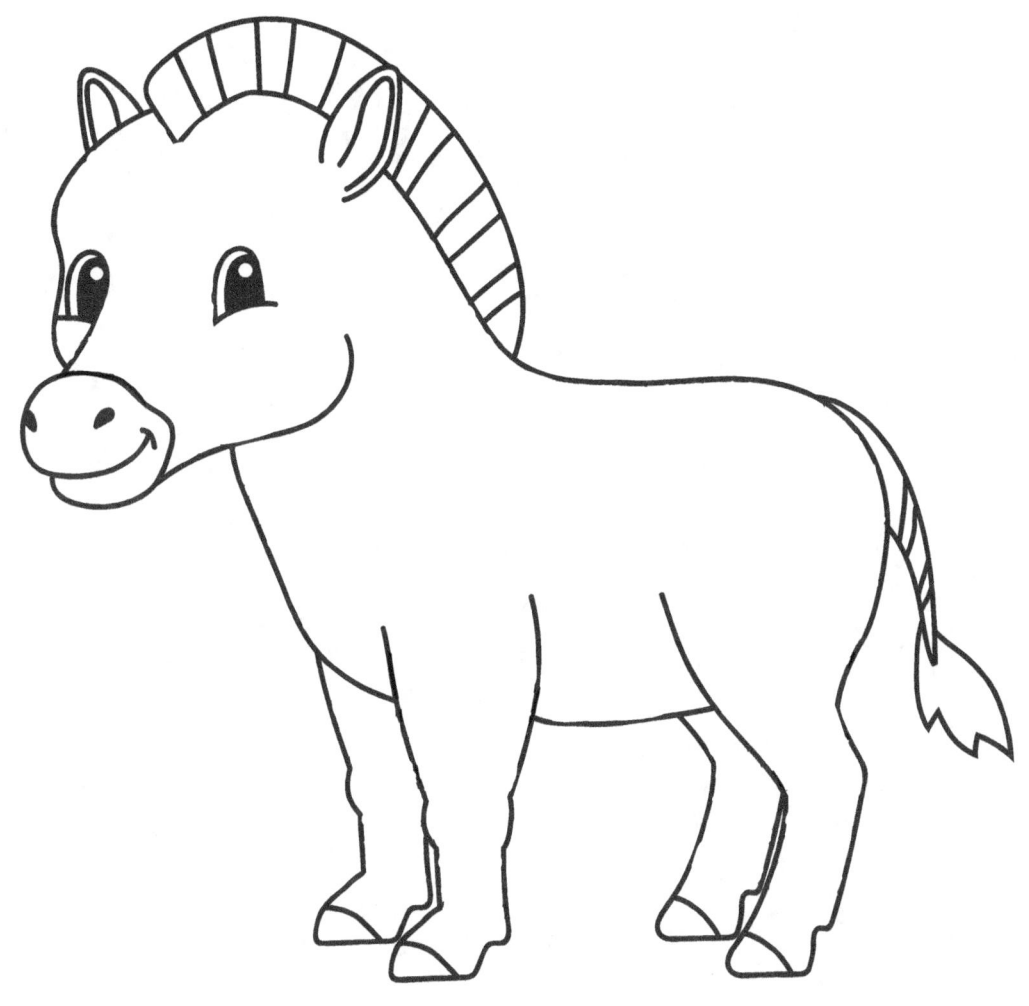

This zebra lost its stripes.

Can you draw them on?

Love for All Creatures

Becoming a vet means having a big heart for all creatures, big and small

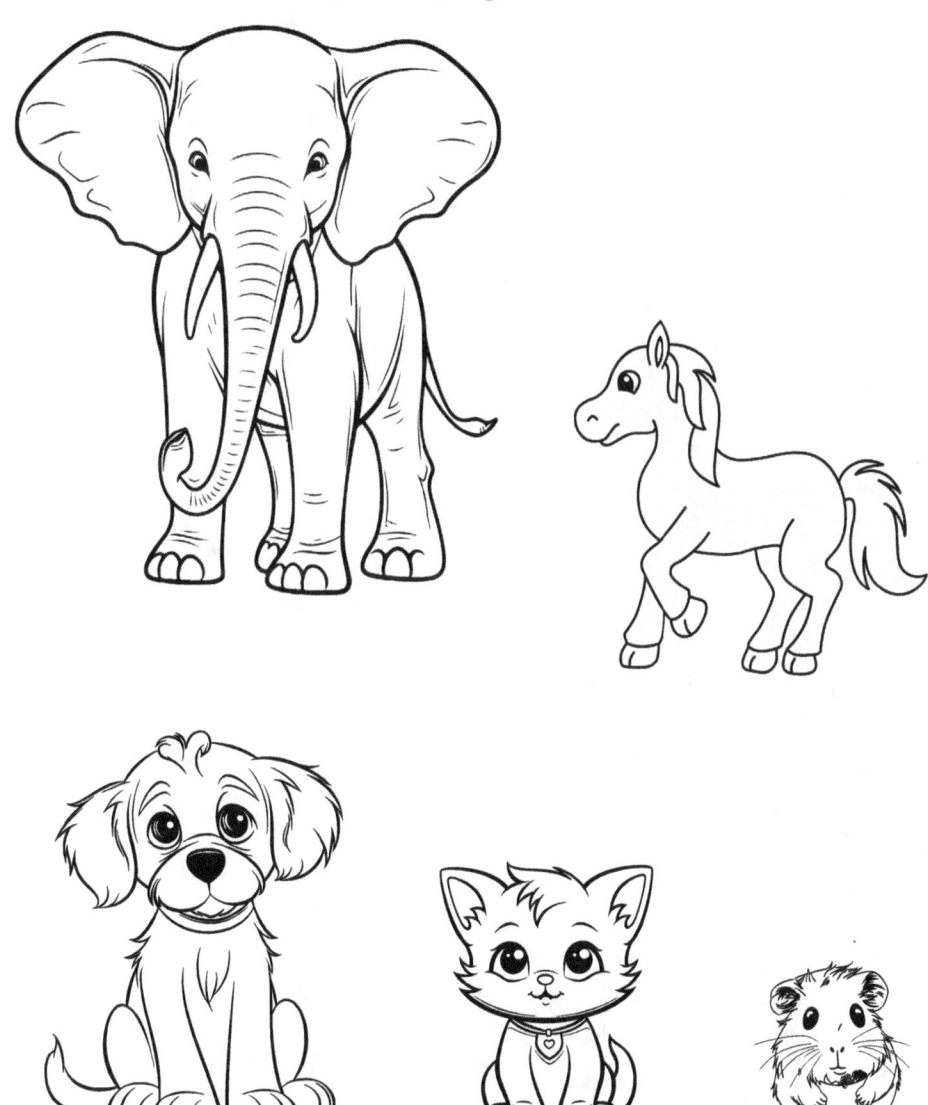

Dream Big

If you love animals, dream big – you could be a fantastic veterinarian and make the world a better place for our furry friends!

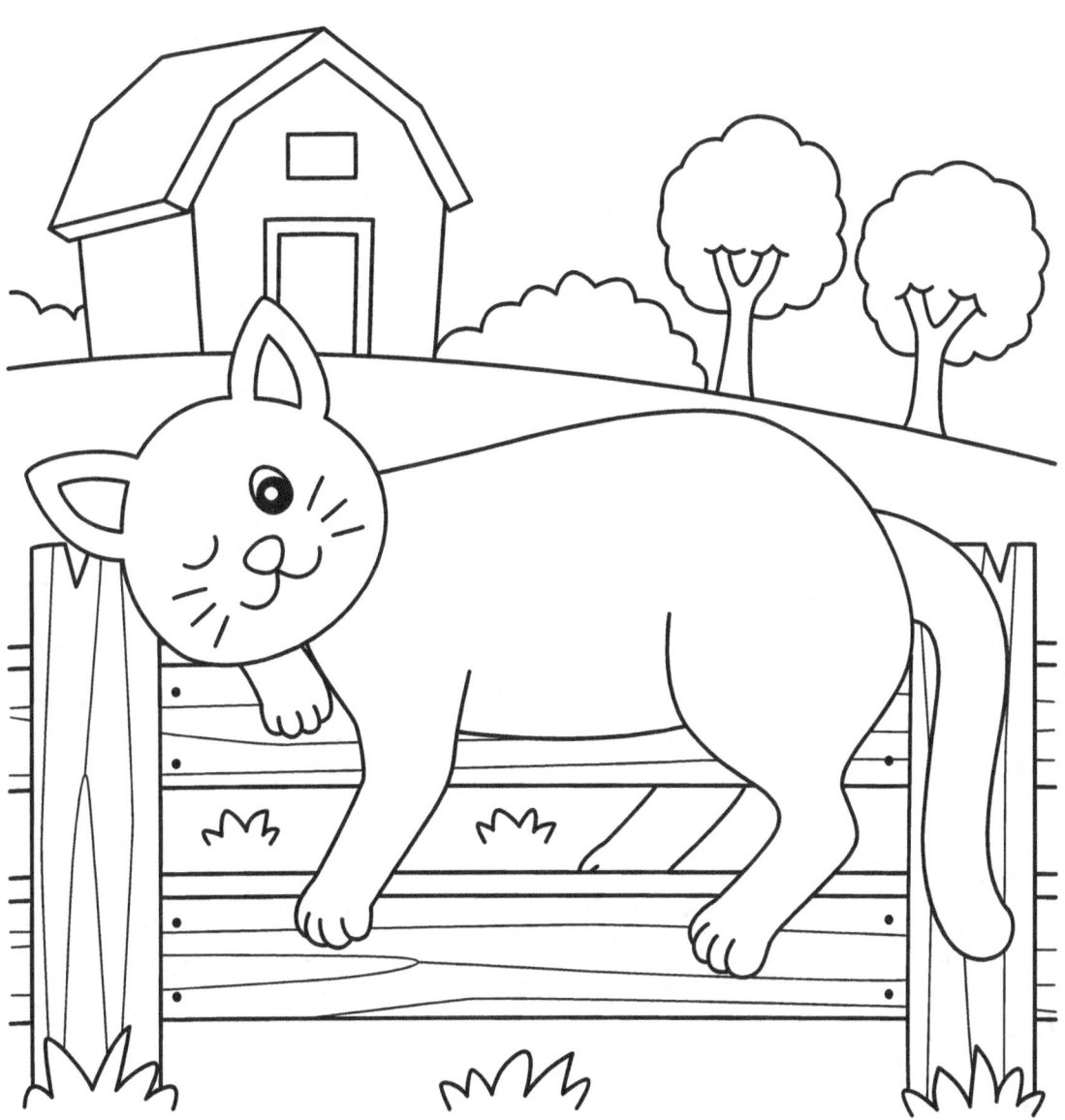